Second Edition

Certification Logbook for Competencies in Clinical Physiology Procedures

for Phase I M.B.B.S Students

(As per Latest CBME Curriculum of Board of Governors, MCI)

Student's Name: _____ S/D/O Sh. _____

Name of College: _____

Date of admission to MBBS course: _____

Date of beginning of Phase I: _____

College Roll No.: _____ University Roll No.: _____

Permanent Address: _____

_____

E-mail ID (Optional): _____

*Certified that the above candidate has **satisfactorily completed/not completed** all the 13 Clinical Physiology competencies mentioned in this logbook for Phase I MBBS. He/she is **eligible/ineligible** to appear for the final University examinations as on date mentioned below.*

_____
(Signature of Faculty In-charge,
Department of Physiology)

_____
(Signature of Professor and Head,
Department of Physiology)

Date: _____

Second Edition

Certification Logbook for Competencies in Clinical Physiology Procedures

for Phase I MBBS Students

(As per Latest CBME Curriculum of Board of Governors, MCI)

Compiled by

Jyoti Sethi MBBS MD
Dean Academics Cum
Professor and Head
Department of Physiology
Kalpana Chawla Government Medical College
Karnal, Haryana, India

Sharat Gupta MBBS MD
Professor
Department of Physiology
Kalpana Chawla Government Medical College
Karnal, Haryana, India

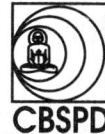

CBSPD

CBS Publishers & Distributors Pvt Ltd

New Delhi • Bengaluru • Chennai • Kochi • Kolkata • Lucknow • Mumbai
Hyderabad • Jharkhand • Nagpur • Patna • Pune • Uttarakhand

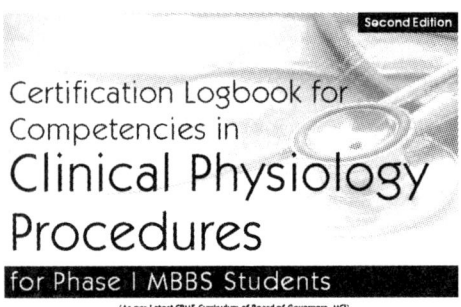

Second Edition

Certification Logbook for Competencies in
Clinical Physiology Procedures
for Phase I MBBS Students
(As per Latest CBME Curriculum of Board of Governors, MCI)

ISBN: 978-81-947082-2-3

Copyright © Authors and Publisher

Second Edition: 2021
Reprint: 2022, 2023, 2024, 2025
First Edition: 2020

Published by Satish Kumar Jain and produced by Varun Jain for

CBS Publishers & Distributors Pvt Ltd
4819/XI Prahlad Street, 24 Ansari Road, Daryaganj, New Delhi 110 002, India.
Ph: 011-23289259, 23266838
Website: www.cbspd.com
e-mail: delhi@cbspd.com
Corporate Office: 204 FIE, Industrial Area, Patparganj, Delhi 110 092
Ph: 011-4934 4934   Fax: 011-4934 4935   e-mail: publishing@cbspd.com; publicity@cbspd.com

Branches

- **Bengaluru:** Seema House 2975, 17th Cross, K.R. Road, Banasankari 2nd Stage, Bengaluru 560 070, Karnataka, India
  Ph: +91-80-26771678/79   Fax: +91-80-26771680   e-mail: bangalore@cbspd.com
- **Chennai:** 7, Subbaraya Street, Shenoy Nagar, Chennai 600 030, Tamil Nadu, India
  Ph: +91-44-26680620/26681266   Fax: +91-44-42032115   e-mail: chennai@cbspd.com
- **Kochi:** 42/1325, 1326, Power House Road, Opp KSEB, Ernakulam 682 018, Kochi, Kerala, India
  Ph: +91-484-4059061-65, 67   Fax: +91-484-4059065   e-mail: kochi@cbspd.com
- **Kolkata:** 147, Hind Ceramics Compound, 1st Floor, Nilgunj road, Belghoria, Kolkata 700056, West Bengal, India
  Ph: 033-25633055/56   e-mail: kolkata@cbspd.com
- **Lucknow:** Basement, Khushnuma Complex, 7-Meerabai Marg (Behind Jawahar Bhawan), Lucknow-226 001, Uttar Pradesh, India.
  Ph: +0552-4000032   e-mail:tiwari.lucknowi@cbspd.com
- **Mumbai:** PWD shed, Gala No. 25/26, Ramchandra Bhatt Marg, Next to JJ Hospital Gate No. 2, OPP, Union Bank of India, Noorbaug, Mumbai-400009, Maharashtra, India
  Ph: 022-66661880/89   e-mail: mumbai@cbspd.com

Representatives

• **Hyderabad**	0-9885175004	• **Jharkhand**	0-9811541605	• **Nagpur**	0-8692091830
• **Patna**	0-9334159340	• **Pune**	0-9664372571	• **Uttarakhand**	0-9716462459

Printed at SRK Graphics, Delhi, India

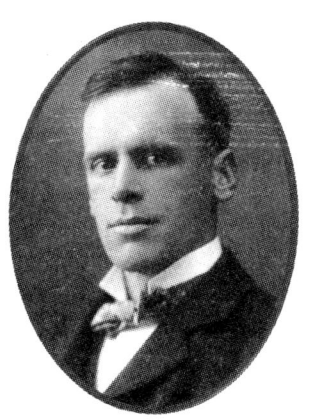

"Physiology of today is the medicine of tomorrow"
Dr Earnest Henry Starling
British Physiologist
(1866–1927)

Foreword

It gives me immense pleasure in writing the Foreword to this *manual Certification Logbook for Competencies in Clinical Physiology Procedures* authored by Prof Jyoti Sethi and Associate Prof Dr Sharat Gupta, Department of Physiology, Kalpana Chawla Government Medical College, Karnal. In 2014, I co-authored an article in *Medical Teachers* on **Medical Education in India: Current Challenges and the Way Forward.** We had emphasized the role of skill development during teaching and training of the medical students of India. I am happy to note that new curriculum brought out by the Board of Governors of Medical Council of India has given ample emphasis for Competency Based Medical Education (CBME). The new curriculum has been restructured and introduced from the academic year of 2019–20.

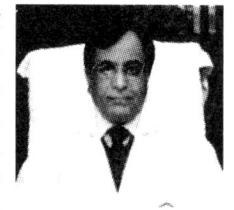

Physiology teaching during the undergraduate trainings as per CBME required 13 procedures to be perfected by each MBBS student needing certification by the Head, Department of Physiology, at the end of the session. To fulfil this requirement this manual will ensure quantification and assessment of students in clinical physiology in an objective and standardized manner leaving no chance of subjective bias. Further, the checklist for each procedure based on objective structured clinical examination (OSCE) has been provided. The assessment card provided in the logbook will facilitate the teacher to evaluate every student in a holistic manner with reference to his/her clinical skills and soft skills as a part of assessment of cognitive as well as communicative (AETCOM) domains.

What is most impressive about this *manual* is that it is comprehensive and as per the CBME requirements. I am sure that both medical teachers as well as students will benefit from the extensive efforts made by Prof Jyoti Sethi and Associate Prof Dr Sharat Gupta in bringing out this book in the shortest possible time.

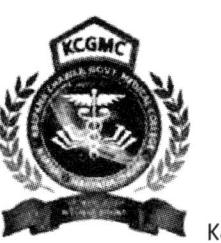

Dr Surender Kashyap

Ex Director
Kalpana Chawla Government Medical College
Karnal, Haryana

Vice Chancellor
Atal Medical and Research University, Mandi (HP)

Foreword

It gives me immense pleasure to write the Foreword to this very useful and helpful *manual* conceptualized and brought out with the objective of standardizing the certification of certain competencies in clinical physiology, by two very dedicated and active teachers who are not only experts in their subject but are also motivated to implement the new CBME curriculum in letter and spirit.

During attending the various faculty development programs, first as a learner in regional/nodal centers and later as a resource faculty in different medical colleges, I observed that there was a lot of apprehension and speculation about the process of certification of competencies during the implementation of CBME curriculum. Nobody actually knew how to go about it and wanted some guidance about it. The common point of concern was as to how uniformity will be attained in various medical colleges across the country. This issue also came up in our discussion when we were preparing the First Prof time table at our institute. We strongly felt a need that there must be a standardization of the certification methods, otherwise it will compromise the essence of CBME. That was the moment when the idea of this *manual* was conceived by the authors and in record time they came out with the manual. Not only the effort but also the purpose is commendable. The USP of this manual is that the certification method has been framed by using reputed international clinical medicine textbooks as a reference.

I am sure this manual will prove to be very helpful for both teachers and students as it will help in reducing the subjective variation in certification and assessment of competencies. I also feel it will provide framework and motivation for designing such a manual for other specialties of the course.

Dr Himanshu Madaan
Medical Superintendent cum Professor
Department of Biohemistry
Kalpana Chawla Govt Medical College, Karnal

Resource Faculty, MCI Regional Centre for
Faculty Development Programs, MAMC
New Delhi

Ex Dean Academics
Kalpana Chawla Government Medical College
Karnal, Haryana

Preface to the Second Edition

The year 2019 proved to be a turning point in the history of medical education since the Board of Governors; Medical Council of India introduced the competency based curriculum for medical undergraduates (CBME). The primary objective of this new curriculum is improvement of clinical skills of the Indian Medical Graduate (IMG) via mandatory certification of certain essential clinical procedures across various disciplines of medicine, including Physiology. The previous edition of this logbook was a maiden venture of the authors in this direction. We received an overwhelming support and constructive comments from our fellow colleagues throughout India who whole-heartedly embraced this book. Based on some of the inputs which we have received and also on the logbook guidelines which were recently issued by the Board of Governors, Medical Council of India (now replaced by National Medical Commission), we have revamped this logbook with a few subtle yet important changes so as to make it more pragmatic. We hope to continue receiving your valuable inputs to improve the future editions also.

Salient features:

1. The layout and format has been revised based on the logbook guidelines issued by Medical Council of India.
2. Index section has been revamped to indicate the no. and type of attempt for a particular procedure.
3. The assessment system for competencies has been modified as per latest recommendations of MCI.
4. Observations/Results obtained by the students for a procedure can be recorded in the ACTIVITY PERFORMA that is provided with each procedure.
5. Checklists for various clinical procedures have been reframed by including important steps and precautions relevant to those procedures.

Jyoti Sethi

Sharat Gupta

Preface to the First Edition

The Board of Governors, Medical Council of India, has recently overhauled the age-old medical curriculum and has recently introduced the Competency Based Undergraduate Curriculum for the Indian medical graduate. This new curriculum has been designed keeping in mind the long pending demand of the experts of removing redundancy from the age-old curriculum and incorporating contemporary methodologies centred on acquisition of clinical skills by the MBBS students right from 1st year itself. It has also been felt that the student should be competent enough in certain basic clinical procedures being taught in the subject of human physiology, so that when they enter clinical ward/OPDs in 2nd year during clinical postings, they should be confident enough in performing basic clinical examination procedures on actual patients. A total of 13 such procedures in clinical physiology have been identified which need to be certified by the Professor and Head, Department of Physiology of medical colleges throughout India, for each student.

In this regard, the present logbook serves a dual purpose. On the one hand, it provides a ready reference which will guide the teachers as to how to assess the student in a holistic manner and on the other, at the same time it will also serve as a record book in which the data pertaining to the student certification and assessment can be entered.

We would also like to appraise our worthy colleagues and students that the contents of this book are open to constructive comments/review/suggestions. We will try to incorporate these in the future editions of this book. It is recommended that both the teachers as well as the students should read the corresponding guidelines given at the beginning of this book so that they can derive maximum benefit from this book.

Jyoti Sethi
Sharat Gupta

Acknowledgements

We bow our heads in gratitude before the Supreme Almighty for bestowing us with the intellect, resources, zeal and good luck; all of which are equally important for the success of any venture.

We are deeply indebted to our teachers who shaped the course of our academic careers with their assiduous pedagogy and meticulous guidance.

We are also grateful to our family members for being our pillar of strength and providing us their much needed love and moral support 24 × 7 during the preparation of this manuscript. Without them, this project would have never seen light of the day.

We extend our thanks to Dr Surender Kashyap, worthy Director, Kalpana Chawla Government Medical College, Karnal, Haryana, for providing a conducive academic environment and motivating us to fulfil his mission of making KCGMC a world class institution.

Our heartfelt gratitude is also due to Dr Himanshu Madaan, Professor of Biochemistry and Dean Academics, Kalpana Chawla Government Medical College, Karnal, Haryana, and Resource Faculty for MCI Regional Centre for Faculty Development Programme, Maulana Azad Medical College, New Delhi. It is her undulating passion in the field of medical education that has constantly motivated us to give our 100% efforts for the success of CBME curriculum.

Most importantly, our heartfelt thanks is also due to the entire team of CBS Publishers, especially Mr Satish Kumar Jain (CMD), Mr Varun Jain (Director), Mr YN Arjuna (Senior Vice President—Publishing, Editorial and Publicity), Mr Sumit Behl (Assistant Marketing Manager) and Ms Ritu Chawla (General Manager) for realising our potential and helping us in fruition of this manuscript.

Last but not the least, we are also thankful to all our students, past and present, because it is their presence that constantly inspires us to do better!

Jyoti Sethi
Sharat Gupta

Contents

Index

Sr. No.	Competency No. and Name of activity addressed	Date on which completed (dd/mm/yy)	Attempt at activity First (F) Repeat (R) Remedial (Re)	Rating Below expectations (B) Meets expectations (M) Exceeds expectations (E)	Decision of faculty Completed (C) Repeat (R) Remedial (R)	Initials of faculty with date	Feedback received Initial of student
	CARDIOVASCULAR SYSTEM *No. of procedures that require certification: 03*						
1.	PY 5.12 Record pulse and blood pressure at rest in a volunteer.		F				
			R1				
			R2				
			Re				
2.	PY 5.12 Record pulse and blood pressure in a volunteer in different grades of exercise.		F				
			R1				
			R2				
			Re				
3.	PY 5.12 Record the blood pressure in a volunteer during change of posture.		F				
			R1				
			R2				
			Re				
	RESPIRATORY SYSTEM *No. of procedures that require certification: 01*						
4.	PY 6.9 Demonstrate the correct clinical examination of respiratory system in a normal volunteer or simulated environment.		F1				
			R1				
			R2				
			Re				
	NEUROPHYSIOLOGY *No. of procedures that require certification: 09*						
5.	PY 10.11 Demonstrate the correct clinical examination of higher functions of nervous system in a normal volunteer or simulated environment.		F				
			R1				
			R2				
			Re				
6.	PY 10.11 Demonstrate the correct clinical examination of sensory system in a normal volunteer or simulated environment.		F1				
			R1				
			R2				
			Re				

Sr. No.	Competency No. and Name of activity addressed	Date on which completed (dd/mm/yy)	Attempt at activity First (F) Repeat (R) Remedial (Re)	Rating Below expectations (B) Meets expectations (M) Exceeds expectations (E)	Decision of faculty Completed (C) Repeat (R) Remedial (R)	Initials of faculty with date	Feedback received Initial of student
7.	PY 10.11 Demonstrate the correct clinical examination of motor system in a normal volunteer or simulated environment.		F				
			R1				
			R2				
			Re				
8.	PY 10.11 Demonstrate the correct clinical examination of reflexes in a normal volunteer or simulated environment.		F				
			R1				
			R2				
			Re				
9.	PY 10.11 Demonstrate the correct clinical examination of cranial nerves in a normal volunteer or simulated environment.		F				
			R1				
			R2				
			Re				
10.	PY 10.20 Demonstrate clinical testing of visual acuity, colour and field of vision in a normal volunteer or simulated environment		F				
			R1				
			R2				
			Re				
11.	PY 10.20 Demonstrate hearing tests in a normal volunteer or simulated environment.		F				
			R1				
			R2				
			Re				
12.	PY 10.20 Demonstrate testing of smell in a normal volunteer or simulated environment.		F				
			R1				
			R2				
			Re				
13.	PY 10.20 Demonstrate taste sensation in a normal volunteer or simulated environment.		F				
			R1				
			R2				
			Re				

How to Use this Certification Logbook
A Guide for Teachers

- The student should initially be given a detailed demonstration of the procedure on a normal subject via DOAP (demonstrate observe assist perform) method.

- The student must then practice that procedure under supervision of a teacher until he/she is confident about performing these procedures independently.

- Thereafter an assessment of the practical skills may be carried out based on the corresponding Objective Structured Clinical Examination (OSCE) pattern. A checklist for the same has been included for stepwise evaluation of each clinical skill. The teachers are required to quantitatively assess the students for each competency.

- The scoring system has been designed to assess the cognitive domain as well as the Attitude, Ethics and Communication (AETCOM) domains of the students.

- Each student will be assessed on a scale of 1–5, separately for the following 5 parameters, i.e. behaviour (towards the subject), communication, confidence level, procedural skills (i.e. systematic approach during the procedure) and knowledge level (i.e. viva voce). In this way each competency will be assessed on a total of 25 points. A suggestive scoring table has been given in the assessment card of each procedure to help the teachers decide the score to be awarded for each skill.

- The cumulative total of the score obtained by the student in these five parameters will then be graded as follows:

Cumulative score	Grading
9 or less	Below Expectations (B)
10–19	Meets Expectations (M)
20 and more	Exceeds Expectations (E)

- A student needs to obtain a minimum final score of 10 (i.e. he/she should Meet Expectations) in each procedure in order to be declared competent and for closure of that procedure. If the student is able to complete the certification for a competency in first attempt, the same is indicated as "F" (i.e. First attempt) in the corresponding column of the index.

- If the student is "Below Expectations" in any activity, he/she should repeat it. The repeat attempt is indicated as "R1 or R2" (i.e. repeat attempt 1 or 2) in the index. If two consecutive repeat attempts are unsuccessful, the faculty should review and discuss the problematic areas with the student and then ask him/her to appear for a remedial attempt, indicated as "Re" in the index. A student who scores "B" grade in remedial attempt will be considered incompetent/unsuccessful in that procedure.

- The teachers should share their feedback on the student's performance after every attempt and indicate the same in the teacher's remarks section of assessment card. This will encourage the student to identify his/her individual strengths as well as weaknesses in each procedure. Whether the student has received any feedback or not should be indicated by writing "Yes/No" in last column of index along with his/her signatures.

- Some longer clinical procedures (e.g. examination of cranial nerves, examination of reflexes, etc.) may be conducted in more than one session taken on consecutive days. However, the closure of such certification(s) should be done only at the end of the final session for that procedure.

- Upon successful completion of all the 13 procedures, the faculty in-charge MBBS from the concerned physiology department of that institution will issue a COMPLETION CERTIFICATE to each student which shall be counter-signed by the Professor and Head of that Physiology Department and also by the Principal/Dean of that institute. The template for the same is also provided in this logbook. The completed logbooks will be retained by the department for record purposes.

- **Note:** The students will maintain a written record of their activities and performance during that procedure. For this purpose, predesigned ACTIVITY PERFORMAS specific for each clinical procedure have been provided in this logbook. Their contents have been standardised and prepared from the following internationally renowned clinical textbooks:

1. *Bates' Guide to Physical Examination and History Taking.* 12th edition. Lynn S Bickley. Wolters Kluwer Publishers.

2. *Hutchinson's Clinical Methods: An Integrated Approach to Clinical Practice.* 24th edition. Elsevier Publishers.

3. *Macleod's Clinical Examination.* 13th edition. Churchill Livingstone Publishers.

Thank You!

How to Perform Well in Competency Assessment
Some Tips for Students

- **General tips:**
  1. Dress appropriately; formal wear is the best.
  2. ALWAYS wear your apron.
  3. Listen carefully to your examiner and try to answer with politeness, confidence and common sense. DO NOT argue at any point.
  4. Be confident; BUT don't be overconfident or underconfident.

- **Approach towards the subject/patient:**
  1. ALWAYS GREET the subject before starting the procedure.
  2. Be sure to obtain subject's consent (written/verbal) prior to examination.
  3. It is advisable to converse with subject in his/her local language and know his name, age, background, job, etc. before you start the procedure. This will help you in developing a good rapport with the subject and ensure his/her cooperation during the procedure.
  4. Be very clear while giving instructions to your subject and also explain him/her the procedure in brief. Try not to seem confused.
  5. Before performing any procedure, be sure to crosscheck that he/she has fully understood the same. DON'T START the procedure until you are ABSOLUTELY SURE that he/she has understood your instructions.
  6. Stop the procedure at any point if you feel that the subject is feeling uneasy or uncomfortable. Reassure him/her and restart.
  7. Always thank your subject at the end of the procedure.

- **Methodology:**
  1. Before starting the examination, ensure that you have all the necessary equipment and it is in working condition.
  2. Always remember "The eye sees what the mind knows"; thus it is important that you should always plan the steps beforehand and then perform the required steps in a proper sequence so that you don't miss any of the steps.
  3. You should have "a damsel's hand (firm yet gentle) and an aquiline (eagle like) vision" during the procedure.

- **Data compilation and presentation of results:**
  1. Record the observations and express the results in proper units.
  2. Document your findings in a neat and tidy manner. It is better to avoid cutting and overwriting as much as possible.
  3. For final result/interpretation purpose, the student should compare the findings/values obtained in the subject with the standard parameters.
  4. The final result should always be reported in a proper format.
     - *For example, the result for BP may be given as follows:*
       The BP of the given subject is … mmHg and it is within normal limits/abnormally high/abnormally low.

Good Luck!

CARDIOVASCULAR SYSTEM

PROCEDURE 1

AIM: PY 5.12: Record pulse and blood pressure at rest in a volunteer.

Number of times this skill needs to be done to be certified for independent performance = 01.

Sr. No.	Steps to be performed sequentially	Performed (Y/N)
	Checklist for examination of radial pulse	
i.	Stands on the right side of the subject and explains the procedure in subject's own language.	
ii.	Supports the subject's right arm and holds it in semi-prone and semi-flexed position.	
iii.	Places his/her index, middle and ring fingers on the radial artery of the subject.	
iv.	Counts the pulse rate for 1 full minute.	
v.	Determines other important characteristics of pulse.	
vi.	Expresses the result in proper format.	
	Checklist for arterial blood pressure (BP)	
i.	Stands on the right side of the subject and explains the procedure in subject's own language.	
ii.	Checks the BP apparatus for any zero error and/or leakage in mercury bulb or cuff.	
iii.	Keeps the BP apparatus at the level of the heart.	
iv.	Exposes the arm up to the shoulder or ensures bare minimum clothing on arm.	
v.	Wraps the BP cuff firmly around the upper arm, keeping its lower edge 2.5 cm above antecubital crease. Checks that it is snugly fit.	
vi.	Performs palpatory method first and notes the reading.	
vii.	Re-inflates the cuff and raises the mercury column around 30 mmHg more than the reading obtained by palpatory method.	
viii.	Performs auscultatory method.	
ix.	Takes 3 separate readings of SBP and DBP at 2 minutes intervals and takes their average to obtain final reading.	
x.	Expresses the result in proper format.	

ACTIVITY PERFORMA FOR PROCEDURE 1

(use Xerox copy for Repeat/Remedial attempts)

Subject's name: Date:

Age:

Gender: Male/Female

Observations:

Examination of radial pulse:

Rate:	_____ per minute.
Rhythm:	Regularly regular/regularly irregular/irregularly irregular.
Volume:	Good/Low/High
Character:	No special character/_____ *(specify if any special character is present)*
Condition of vessel wall:	Palpable/Not palpable
Equality on both sides:	Equal/Unequal
Radiofemoral delay:	Present/Absent
Other peripheral pulses:	Palpable/_____(specify if non-palpable)

*(*Ulnar, Brachial, Carotid, Popliteal, Tibial, Dorsalis Pedis, etc.)*

Recording of BP:

Zero error in instrument (if any): _____

Palpatory method: Systolic BP: _____ mmHg.

Auscultatory method:

	Reading 1*	Reading 2*	Reading 3*
Systolic BP (mmHg)			
Diastolic BP (mmHg)			

*(*Deduct zero error from above readings, if present)*

Result/Interpretation:

Signature of student   **Signature of teacher**

*Note:

Blood pressure classification for adults as per JNC 7 guidelines of American Society of Hypertension.

Category	Systolic BP (mmHg)	Diastolic BP (mmHg)
Normal	<120	<80
Prehypertension	120–139	80–89
Stage 1 hypertension	140–159	90–99
Stage 2 hypertension	≥160	≥100

Ref: https://www.nhlbi.nih.gov/files/docs/guidelines/jnc7full.pdf

ASSESSMENT CARD FOR PROCEDURE 1*

Type of Attempt *(please tick)*: **First/Repeat 1/Repeat 2/Remedial**
(use Xerox copy for Repeat/Remedial attempts)

Sr. No.	Attributes to be assessed	Score (1–5)*
i.	Behavioural skill	
ii.	Communication skill	
iii.	Confidence level	
iv.	Procedural skill	
v.	Knowledge level	
	Cumulative total (out of 25)	

*Note: The teacher may decide the score as given below:

Below average	Average	Good	Very good	Excellent
1	2	3	4	5

Grading of candidate (please tick): **B / M / E**

Cumulative total	Grading
9 or less	Below Expectations (B)
10–19	Meets Expectations (M)
20 and above	Exceeds Expectations (E)

Teacher's feedback:

_____

_____

_____

_____

_____

Signature of teacher (with date)

PROCEDURE 2

AIM: PY 5.12 Record pulse and blood pressure in a volunteer in different grades of exercise.

Number of times this skill needs to be done to be certified for independent performance = 01.

	Checklist for procedure	
Sr. No.	*Steps to be performed sequentially*	*Performed (Y/N)*
i.	Notes the subject's age to determine the maximum heart rate and the target heart rate (to be achieved) as per the intensity of exercise to be performed.	
ii.	Stands on the right side of the subject and explains the procedure in subject's own language.	
iii.	Checks the BP apparatus for any zero error and/or leakage in mercury bulb or cuff.	
iv.	Asks the subject to observe complete mental and physical rest for at least 5 minutes.	
v.	Keeps BP apparatus at the level of the heart and records the pulse and BP of the subject at rest.	
vi.	Without removing the BP cuff, asks the subject to perform exercise of pre-determined intensity (i.e. mild/moderate or severe).	
vii.	Records the pulse and BP immediately after exercise.	
viii.	Records the pulse and BP after 5 minutes of exercise.	
ix.	Records the pulse and BP again after 10 minutes of exercise.	
x.	Compares the pre- and post-exercise pulse and BP values and expresses the result in proper format.	

ACTIVITY PERFORMA FOR PROCEDURE 2

(use Xerox copy for Repeat/Remedial attempts)

Subject's name: Date:

Age:

Gender: Male/Female

Observations:

Intensity of exercise:*   Mild/Moderate/Severe

	Pulse rate (beats per minute)	Blood pressure (mmHg)	
		Systolic	Diastolic
At rest (baseline values)			
Immediately after exercise			
5 minutes after exercise			
10 minutes after exercise			

Result/Interpretation:

Signature of student   **Signature of teacher**

*Intensity of exercise to be decided as per guidelines given by American Heart Association as follows:

1. Calculate the Maximum Heart Rate (MHR) of the subject using the following formula:

MHR = 220 – age (in years)

2. Intensity of the exercise can then be gauged from the following table

Heart rate at the end of exercise	Exercise intensity
<50% of MHR	Mild
50–70% of MHR	Moderate
>70% of MHR	Severe

Source: Official website of American Heart Association:

https://www.heart.org/en/healthy-living/fitness/fitness-basics/target-heart-rates

ASSESSMENT CARD FOR PROCEDURE 2*

Type of Attempt *(please tick)*: First/Repeat 1/Repeat 2/Remedial
(use Xerox copy for Repeat/Remedial attempts)

Sr. No.	Attributes to be assessed	Score (1–5)*
i.	Behavioural skill	
ii.	Communication skill	
iii.	Confidence level	
iv.	Procedural skill	
v.	Knowledge level	
	Cumulative total (out of 25)	

*Note: The teacher may decide the score as given below:

Below average	Average	Good	Very good	Excellent
1	2	3	4	5

Grading of candidate *(please tick)*: **B / M / E**

Cumulative total	Grading
9 or less	Below Expectations (B)
10–19	Meets Expectations (M)
20 and above	Exceeds Expectations (E)

Teacher's feedback:

_____

_____

_____

_____

_____

Signature of teacher (with date)

PROCEDURE 3

AIM: PY 5.12 Record the blood pressure in a volunteer during change of posture.

Number of times this skill needs to be done to be certified for independent performance = 01.

Sr. No.	Steps to be performed sequentially	Performed (Y/N)
	Checklist for procedure	
i.	Stands on the right side of the subject and explains the procedure in subject's own language.	
ii.	Checks the BP apparatus for any zero error and/or leakage in mercury bulb or cuff.	
iii.	Asks the patient to lie down supine on a couch.	
iv.	Keeps BP apparatus at the level of the heart.	
v.	Records BP by both palpatory and auscultatory methods.	
vi.	Without removing the BP cuff, asks the subject to stand up quickly without support.	
vii.	Records BP immediately upon standing.	
viii.	Records BP again after 3 minutes of standing.	
ix.	Compares the BP values in supine and standing posture and expresses the results in proper format.	

ACTIVITY PERFORMA FOR PROCEDURE 3

(use Xerox copy for Repeat/Remedial attempts)

Subject's name: Date:

Age:

Gender: Male/Female

Observations:

	Blood Pressure (mmHg)	
	Systolic	*Diastolic*
Supine posture		
Immediately upon standing		
3 minutes after standing		

Result/Interpretation:

Signature of student   **Signature of teacher**

ASSESSMENT CARD FOR PROCEDURE 3*

Type of Attempt (please tick): First/Repeat 1/Repeat 2/Remedial
(use Xerox copy for Repeat/Remedial attempts)

Sr. No.	Attributes to be assessed	Score (1–5)*
i.	Behavioural skill	
ii.	Communication skill	
iii.	Confidence level	
iv.	Procedural skill	
v.	Knowledge level	
	Cumulative total (out of 25)	

Note: The teacher may decide the score as given below:

Below average	Average	Good	Very good	Excellent
1	2	3	4	5

Grading of candidate (please tick): **B / M / E**

Cumulative total	Grading
9 or less	Below Expectations (B)
10–19	Meets Expectations (M)
20 and above	Exceeds Expectations (E)

Teacher's feedback:

_____

_____

_____

_____

_____

Signature of teacher (with date)

RESPIRATORY SYSTEM

PROCEDURE 4

AIM: PY 6.9 Demonstrate the correct clinical examination of respiratory system in a normal volunteer or simulated environment.

Number of times this skill needs to be done to be certified for independent performance = 01.

\multicolumn{3}{c}{Checklist for procedure}		
Sr. No.	*Steps to be performed sequentially*	*Performed (Y/N)*
i.	Stands on the right side of the subject and explains the procedure briefly in subject's own language.	
ii.	Takes a brief and relevant history of the patient before starting the physical examination.	
iii.	Performs the general physical examination of the patient.	
iv.	Starts with inspection of thorax and looks for: a. Shape of the chest b. Movement of chest c. Breathing pattern d. Visible scar mark (if any)	
v.	Palpates the thorax to note: a. Local temperature b. Tenderness (if any) c. Position of trachea d. Chest expansion e. Vocal fremitus	
vi.	Performs percussion of thorax to note: a. Chest resonance b. Cardiac dullness c. Liver dullness	
vii.	Auscultates the thorax to note: a. Type of breath sounds b. Presence/absence of adventitious sounds c. Vocal resonance	
viii.	Records the findings in a proper format.	

ACTIVITY PERFORMA FOR PROCEDURE 4

(use Xerox copy for Repeat/Remedial attempts)

Subject's name: Date:

Age:

Gender: Male/Female

Occupation:

Non-smoker/Chronic smoker/Occasional smoker *(please tick)*

Brief relevant history:

General physical examination:

Pallor:	Present/Absent
Icterus:	Present/Absent
Cyanosis:	Present/Absent
Clubbing:	Present/Absent
Lymphadenopathy (cervical/axillary)	Present/Absent

Vitals:

Temperature:	_____°F
Pulse rate:	_____ per min.
BP:	_____ mmHg.
Respiratory rate:	_____ per min.

Respiratory System Examination

INSPECTION

Shape of chest: Normal/abnormal (specify)

Movement of chest: Symmetrical/asymmetrical

Type of breathing: Abdomino-throacic/thoraco-abdominal

Any visible veins/scar mark on chest: No/Yes

PALPATION

Local temperature: Normal/raised

Any area of tenderness: No/Yes (specify)

Position of trachea: Midline/_____ sided

Chest expansion: _____ cm

Vocal fremitus: Normal/Increased/Decreased

PERCUSSION

Chest resonance: Non-resonant/resonant/hyperresonant

Liver dullness: Starts from _____ right intercostal space/absent

Cardiac dullness: Starts from _____ left intercostal space/absent

AUSCULTATION

Breath sounds: Vesicular/Bronchial

Adventitious sounds: Absent/Present (specify type and location)

Vocal resonance: Normal/Increased/Decreased

Result/Interpretation:

Signature of student   **Signature of teacher**

ASSESSMENT CARD FOR PROCEDURE 4*

Type of Attempt (please tick): First/Repeat 1/Repeat 2/Remedial
(use Xerox copy for Repeat/Remedial attempts)

Sr. No.	Attributes to be assessed	Score (1–5)*
i.	Behavioural skill	
ii.	Communication skill	
iii.	Confidence level	
iv.	Procedural skill	
v.	Knowledge level	
	Cumulative total (out of 25)	

*Note: The teacher may decide the score as given below:

Below average	Average	Good	Very good	Excellent
1	2	3	4	5

Grading of candidate (please tick): **B / M / E**

Cumulative total	Grading
9 or less	Below Expectations (B)
10–19	Meets Expectations (M)
20 and above	Exceeds Expectations (E)

Teacher's feedback:

_____

_____

_____

_____

_____

Signature of teacher (with date)

NEUROPHYSIOLOGY

PROCEDURE 5

AIM: PY 10.11 Demonstrate the correct clinical examination of higher functions of nervous system in a normal volunteer or simulated environment.

Number of times this skill needs to be done to be certified for independent performance = 01.

Sr. No.	Steps to be performed sequentially	Performed (Y/N)
	Checklist for procedure	
i.	Makes the patient feel relaxed and comfortable and explains the procedure in subject's own language.	
ii.	Notes the consciousness level of the subject.	
iii.	Notes the general appearance of the subject.	
iv.	Observes the subject's behaviour.	
v.	Observes the subject's emotional state	
vi.	Checks the subject's orientation levels with respect to time, place and person.	
vii.	Observes the presence/absence of any illusion/delusion/hallucination	
viii.	Gauges the memory of subject for recent and past events.	
ix.	Estimates the intelligence level of the subject.	
x.	Observes the speech and handedness of the subject.	

ACTIVITY PERFORMA FOR PROCEDURE 5

(use Xerox copy for Repeat/Remedial attempts)

Subject's name: Date:

Age:

Gender: Male/Female

Occupation:

Higher Functions Assessment

1. Level of consciousness of subject: Alert/Semi-conscious/Unconscious

2. General appearance: Normal/Abnormal

3. Behaviour: Cooperative/Uncooperative

4. Emotional state: Normal/Agitated/Depressed/Other

5. Orientation to time, place and person: Well-oriented/Disoriented

6. Any illusion/delusion/hallucination: Yes/No

   (Describe if present)

7. Memory (recent and past events):   Normal/Abnormal

8. Intelligence: Normal/Subnormal

9. Speech: Normal/Abnormal

   (Describe the type of abnormality, if present)

10. Handedness: Left handed/Right handed

Result/Interpretation:

Signature of student   **Signature of teacher**

ASSESSMENT CARD FOR PROCEDURE 5*

Type of Attempt *(please tick)*: **First/Repeat 1/Repeat 2/Remedial**
(use Xerox copy for Repeat/Remedial attempts)

Sr. No.	Attributes to be assessed	Score (1–5)*
i.	Behavioural skill	
ii.	Communication skill	
iii.	Confidence level	
iv.	Procedural skill	
v.	Knowledge level	
	Cumulative total (out of 25)	

*Note:** The teacher may decide the score as given below:

Below average	Average	Good	Very good	Excellent
1	2	3	4	5

Grading of candidate (please tick): **B / M / E**

Cumulative total	Grading
9 or less	Below Expectations (B)
10–19	Meets Expectations (M)
20 and above	Exceeds Expectations (E)

Teacher's feedback:

_____

_____

_____

_____

_____

Signature of teacher (with date)

PROCEDURE 6

AIM: PY 10.11 Demonstrate the correct clinical examination of sensory system in a normal volunteer or simulated environment.

Number of times this skill needs to be done to be certified for independent performance = 01.

Checklist for procedure		
Sr.No.	*Steps to be performed sequentially*	*Performed (Y/N)*
i.	Stands on the right side of the subject and explains the procedure very clearly in subject's own language.	
ii.	Asks the subject to keep his/her eyes closed throughout the test and turn his/her face towards the opposite side.	
iii.	Performs tests for dorsal column sensations. a. Pressure sensation b. Fine touch c. Proprioception d. Tactile localisation e. Tactile discrimination f. Vibration	
iv.	Performs tests for anterolateral spinothalamic tract sensations. a. Crude touch b. Superficial pain c. Temperature	
v.	Performs tests for synthetic sensations. a. Stereognosis b. Graphesthesia	
vi.	Compares the findings on both sides and records them in a proper format.	

ACTIVITY PERFORMA FOR PROCEDURE 6

(use Xerox copy for Repeat/Remedial attempts)

Subject's name:　　　　　　　　　　　　　　　　Date:

Age:

Gender: Male/Female

Sensory System Assessment

Sensations	Left side	Right side
Dorsal column sensations (perceived/not perceived)		
Pressure		
Fine touch		
Proprioception		
Tactile localisation		
Two-point discrimination		
Vibration		
Anterolateral spinothalamic tract sensations		
Crude touch		
Pain (provide VAS grading)*		
Temperature		
Synthetic sensations		
Stereognosis		
Graphasthesia		

Result/Interpretation:

Signature of student　　　　　　　　　　　　　　　　　　　**Signature of teacher**

*The grading of pain perception should be done as per Visual Analog Scale (VAS). The subject is asked to point out a number to indicate the intensity of pain felt from the scale below:

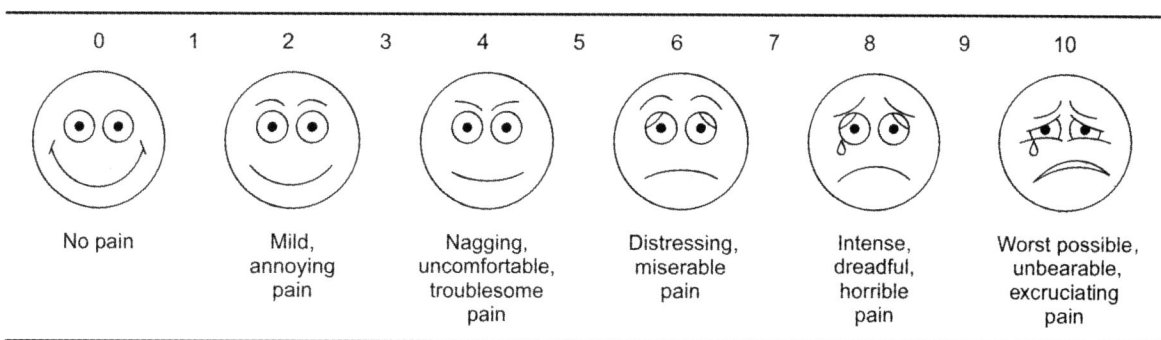

Source: https://operativeneurosurgery.com/doku.php?id=visual_analog_scale

ASSESSMENT CARD FOR PROCEDURE 6*

Type of Attempt *(please tick)*: **First/Repeat 1/Repeat 2/Remedial**
(use Xerox copy for Repeat/Remedial attempts)

Sr. No.	Attributes to be assessed	Score (1–5)*
i.	Behavioural skill	
ii.	Communication skill	
iii.	Confidence level	
iv.	Procedural skill	
v.	Knowledge level	
	Cumulative total (out of 25)	

*Note: The teacher may decide the score as given below:

Below average	Average	Good	Very good	Excellent
1	2	3	4	5

Grading of candidate (please tick): **B / M / E**

Cumulative total	Grading
9 or less	Below Expectations (B)
10–19	Meets Expectations (M)
20 and above	Exceeds Expectations (E)

Teacher's feedback:

_____

_____

_____

_____

_____

Signature of teacher (with date)

PROCEDURE 7

AIM: PY 10.11 Demonstrate the correct clinical examination of motor system in a normal volunteer or simulated environment.

Number of times this skill needs to be done to be certified for independent performance = 01.

	Checklist for procedure	
Sr. No.	*Steps to be performed sequentially*	*Performed (Y/N)*
i.	Stands on the right side of the subject and explains the procedure very clearly in subject's own language.	
ii.	Asks the subject to expose the limb which is to be examined.	
iii.	Notes the bulk of muscles a. Looks for any obvious sign of muscle wasting or hypertrophy b. Records the mid-arm, mid-thigh and mid-calf circumferences using a measuring tape.	
iv.	Assesses the muscle tone a. In upper limbs b. In lower limbs	
v.	Assesses and grades the strength (power) of muscles a. In upper limbs b. In lower limbs	
vi.	Observes the presence of any involuntary movements.	
vii.	Asks the subject to walk and observes his gait.	
viii.	Compares the observations of upper and lower limbs on both sides and records the findings in proper format.	

ACTIVITY PERFORMA FOR PROCEDURE 7

(use Xerox copy for Repeat/Remedial attempts)

Subject's name: Date:

Age:

Gender: Male/Female

Motor System Examination

Characteristic	Left side	Right side
1. Bulk of muscle		
Muscle wasting/hypertrophy (Y/N)	Upper limb _____ Upper limb _____	Lower limb _____ Lower limb _____
Upper and lower limb circumference		
a. Mid-arm level	Centimeters	Centimeters
b. Mid-thigh level	Centimeters	Centimeters
c. Mid-calf level	Centimeters	Centimeters
2. Muscle tone (normal/hypotonia/hypertonia)		
a. Upper limbs		
b. Lower limbs		
3. Power of muscles (provide grades)*		
a. Hand		
b. Shoulder and arm		
c. Hip and thigh		
d. Leg		
4. Any involuntary movements (Y/N)		
5. Gait of the subject (write Y/N)		
a. Does the subject require support while walking?		
b. Can the subject walk in a straight line without bending sideways?		
c. Can the subject quickly turn around by 180° without losing balance?		
d. Is there any obvious defect in subject's gait?		

Result/Interpretation

1. Bulk of muscle

2. Muscle tone

3. Power of muscles

4. Gait

5. Overall remarks

Signature of student   **Signature of teacher**

* Gradation of muscle power may be done as per Medical Research Council (MRC) scale for muscle strength as follows:

Grade	Description
Grade 0	Complete paralysis.
Grade 1	No movements are possible, only a flicker of contraction is present.
Grade 2	Muscle power can be detected only when effect of gravity is removed by making appropriate postural adjustments.
Grade 3	The limb can be held against gravity but not against passive resistance applied by examiner.
Grade 4	Movements are possible against examiner's resistance; but are weak.
Grade 5	Normal muscle power both against gravity and against examiner's resistance.

Source: http://medicalcriteria.com/web/neuromrc/

ASSESSMENT CARD FOR PROCEDURE 7*

Type of Attempt *(please tick)*: **First/Repeat 1/Repeat 2/Remedial**
(use Xerox copy for Repeat/Remedial attempts)

Sr. No.	Attributes to be assessed	Score (1–5)*
i.	Behavioural skill	
ii.	Communication skill	
iii.	Confidence level	
iv.	Procedural skill	
v.	Knowledge level	
	Cumulative total (out of 25)	

Note: The teacher may decide the score as given below:

Below average	Average	Good	Very good	Excellent
1	2	3	4	5

Grading of candidate (please tick): **B / M / E**

Cumulative total	Grading
9 or less	Below Expectations (B)
10–19	Meets Expectations (M)
20 and above	Exceeds Expectations (E)

Teacher's feedback:

_____

_____

_____

_____

_____

Signature of teacher (with date)

PROCEDURE 8

AIM: PY 10.11 Demonstrate the correct clinical examination of reflexes in a normal volunteer or simulated environment.

Number of times this skill needs to be done to be certified for independent performance = 01.

Sr. No.	Steps to be performed sequentially	Performed (Y/N)
	Checklist for procedure	
i.	Stands on the right side of the subject and explains the procedure very clearly in subject's own language.	
ii.	Asks the subject to relax and sit or lie down and expose the upper/lower limbs and also ensures that the subject is not looking at the procedure.	
iii.	Correctly elicits BICEPS REFLEX (sitting position) a. Flexes the subject's elbow at 90°, semi-pronates his forearm and supports the arm. b. Places his own thumb on subject's biceps tendon and strikes it and observes for contraction of biceps and flexion of elbow.	
iv.	Correctly elicits TRICEPS REFLEX (sitting position) a. Flexes the subject's elbow at 90° and provides support to subject's forearm. b. Strikes the triceps tendon just directly above the olecranon and observes for contraction of triceps and extension of elbow.	
v.	Correctly elicits SUPINATOR REFLEX (sitting position) a. Holds the hand of subject firmly yet lightly as if "shaking hands" and bends the subject's hand in opposite direction to stretch the brachioradialis tendon. b. Strikes the styloid process of the radius and observes for flexion of elbow and supination of forearm	
vi.	Correctly elicits KNEE JERK (sitting position) a. Asks the subject to sit on the edge of the bed or a stool such that the legs can swing freely. b. Asks the subject to keep one knee (to be tested) on the other knee and strikes the patellar tendon and observes for contraction of quadriceps and extension of knee.	
vii.	Correctly elicits ANKLE JERK (supine position) a. Asks the subject to slightly flex and evert the leg (to be tested). b. With one hand, dorsiflexes the foot and strikes the stretched Achilles tendon with other hand and observes for contraction of calf muscles and plantar extension of foot.	
viii.	Correctly elicits JAW JERK a. Asks the subject to partly open the mouth and places his own finger firmly on subject's chin. b. Strikes the finger and observes for immediate closure of mouth (contraction of jaw elevators).	
ix.	Correctly elicits PLANTAR REFLEX (supine position) a. Partially flexes the lower limb of the subject and rotates it externally. b. With left hand grasps subject's leg above ankle and with other hand gently scratches the entire outer edge of the sole with a blunt but pointed object (e.g. tip of a key), starting from the heel and swiftly moving towards the ball of the great toe via lower edge of the metatarsals.	
x.	Asks the patient to perform Jendrassik's manoeuvre in case of non-elicitation of deep tendon reflexes.	
xi.	Compares the results on both sides and records the findings in proper format.	

Important note: This checklist may be customised as per standard protocol being followed by your institute in case the procedure for examination of certain reflexes is different from that described above.

ACTIVITY PERFORMA FOR PROCEDURE 8

(use Xerox copy for Repeat/Remedial attempts)

Subject's name: Date:

Age:

Gender: Male/Female

Reflexes Examination

Reflex	Left side	Right side
Plantar reflex (normal/absent/abnormal)		
Deep reflexes (provide grades for each)*		
Biceps jerk		
Triceps jerk		
Supinator jerk		
Knee jerk		
Ankle jerk		
Jaw jerk		

Result/Interpretation:

Signature of student   **Signature of teacher**

* Reflexes should be graded as follows:

Grade	Written as	Description
0	0	Absent
1	+	Present but weak
2	++	Normal (brisk)
3	+++	Very brisk
4	++++	Clonus

Source: *Bates' Guide to Physical Examination and History Taking*, 12th edition, pp. 758, 773.

Important note: Jendrassik's (reinforcement) manoeuvre, if performed, should be indicated by mentioning "elicited with reinforcement" alongside the grade of the reflex for which it was done.

ASSESSMENT CARD FOR PROCEDURE 8*

Type of Attempt *(please tick)*: **First/Repeat 1/Repeat 2/Remedial**
(use Xerox copy for Repeat/Remedial attempts)

Sr. No.	Attributes to be assessed	Score (1–5)*
i.	Behavioural skill	
ii.	Communication skill	
iii.	Confidence level	
iv.	Procedural skill	
v.	Knowledge level	
	Cumulative total (out of 25)	

*Note:** The teacher may decide the score as given below:

Below average	Average	Good	Very good	Excellent
1	2	3	4	5

Grading of candidate (please tick): **B / M / E**

Cumulative total	Grading
9 or less	Below Expectations (B)
10–19	Meets Expectations (M)
20 and above	Exceeds Expectations (E)

Teacher's feedback:

_____

_____

_____

_____

_____

Signature of teacher (with date)

PROCEDURE 9

AIM: PY 10.11 Demonstrate the correct clinical examination of cranial nerves in a normal volunteer or simulated environment.

Number of times this skill needs to be done to be certified for independent performance = 01.

Sr. No.	Steps to be performed sequentially	Performed (Y/N)
	Checklist for procedure	
i.	Stands on the right side of the subject and explains the procedure very clearly in subject's own language.	
	Checklist for Cranial Nerve I	
i	Performs tests for olfaction.	
	Checklist for Cranial Nerve II	
i.	Checks for acuity of distant and near vision.	
ii.	Performs tests for colour vision.	
iii.	Checks field of vision.	
	Checklist for Cranial Nerves III, IV and VI	
i.	Checks the functioning of extraocular muscles.	
ii.	Elicits direct and indirect light reflex.	
iii.	Elicits accommodation reflex.	
	Checklist for Cranial Nerve V	
i.	Elicits corneal and conjunctival reflexes.	
ii.	Checks muscles of mastication.	
	Checklist for Cranial Nerve VII	
i.	Elicits the motor functions of facial nerve.	
ii.	Elicits the sensory (taste) function of facial nerve.	
	Checklist for Cranial Nerve VIII	
i.	Performs hearing tests.	
	Checklist for Cranial Nerves IX and X	
i.	Elicits palatal and pharyngeal reflexes.	
ii.	Checks for taste sensation on posterior 1/3rd of tongue	
iii.	Asks for history of nasal regurgitation of food from subject.	
	Checklist for Cranial Nerve XI	
i.	Asks the subject to flex his chin against resistance.	
ii.	Asks the subject to shrug his shoulders against resistance.	
	Checklist for Cranial Nerve XII	
i.	Observes for any sign of tongue atrophy and tongue deviation on protrusion	
ii.	Checks the movements of tongue.	

ACTIVITY PERFORMA FOR PROCEDURE 9

(use Xerox copy for Repeat/Remedial attempts)

Subject's name: Date:

Age:

Gender: Male/Female

Cranial Nerves (CN) Examination

(Result to be reported as normal/abnormal or present/absent as appropriate)

Tests performed	Left side	Right side
Olfactory nerve (CN I)*		
i. Smell sensitivity		
Optic nerve (CN II)*		
i. Visual acuity		
ii. Colour vision		
iii. Field of vision		
Occulomotor, trochlear and abducent nerves (CN III, IV and VI)		
i. Pupil (size, shape)		
ii. Ptosis, squint		
iii. Ocular movements		
iv. Pupillary light reflexes		
v. Accommodation reflex		
Trigeminal nerve (CN V)		
i. Corneal and conjunctival reflexes		
ii. Mandibular reflex (muscles of mastication)		
Facial nerve (CN VII)		
i. Facial appearance		
ii. Taste sensation (anterior 2/3rds of tongue)		
iii. Muscles of face		
Vestibulocochlear nerve (CN VIII): Cochlear division*		
i. Hearing tests		
Glossopharyngeal and vagus nerves (CN IX and X)		
i. Palatal and pharyngeal reflexes (CN IX and X)		
ii. Taste sensation on posterior 1/3rd of tongue (CN IX)		
iii. History of nasal regurgitation of food		

Spinal accessory nerve (CN XI)		
i. Flexion of head against resistance		
ii. Rotation of chin		
iii. Shrugging of shoulder		
Hypoglossal nerve (CN XII)		
i. Atrophy of tongue		
ii. Deviation of tongue on protrusion		
iii. Tongue movements		

Important note: OSCE assessment of cranial nerves I, II and VIII can be done concurrently while doing OSCE assessment for procedure 13 (testing of smell), procedure 10 (testing of visual acuity, colour vision and field of vision) and procedure 11 (hearing tests) respectively.

Result/Interpretation:

Signature of student   **Signature of teacher**

ASSESSMENT CARD FOR PROCEDURE 9*
Type of Attempt *(please tick)*: **First/Repeat 1/Repeat 2/Remedial**
(use Xerox copy for Repeat/Remedial attempts)

Sr. No.	Attributes to be assessed	Score (1–5)*
i.	Behavioural skill	
ii.	Communication skill	
iii.	Confidence level	
iv.	Procedural skill	
v.	Knowledge level	
	Cumulative total (out of 25)	

*Note: The teacher may decide the score as given below:

Below average	Average	Good	Very good	Excellent
1	2	3	4	5

Grading of candidate (please tick): **B / M / E**

Cumulative total	Grading
9 or less	Below Expectations (B)
10–19	Meets Expectations (M)
20 and above	Exceeds Expectations (E)

Teacher's feedback:

_____

_____

_____

_____

Signature of teacher (with date)

PROCEDURE 10

AIM: PY 10.20 Demonstrate clinical testing of visual acuity, colour and field of vision in a normal volunteer or simulated environment.

Number of times this skill needs to be done to be certified for independent performance = 01.

Sr. No.	Steps to be performed sequentially	Performed (Y/N)
	Checklist for procedure	
i.	Explains the procedure to the subject in his/her own language.	
ii.	Asks the subject to close opposite eye during the test.	
iii.	Tests the distant vision of the subject.	
	a. Chooses appropriate Snellen's charts as per literacy levels of subject (English chart/Hindi chart/ E-chart/Landolt's ring chart). b. Asks the subject to read out the alphabets while standing at a distance of 6 metres away from the chart.	
iv.	Tests the near vision of the subject.	
	a. Chooses appropriate Jaeger's charts. b. Asks the subject to read the charts from a comfortable reading distance (25 cm).	
v.	Tests the colour vision of the subject.	
	a. Keeps the Ishihara's plates 75 cm away from test eye, perpendicular to the line of sight. b. Makes the subject read out initial 21 plates.	
vi.	Performs confrontation test first for visual field.	
vii.	Charts field of vision by doing perimetry.	
viii.	Compares the result on both sides and reports the observations in proper format.	

ACTIVITY PERFORMA FOR PROCEDURE 10

(use Xerox copy for Repeat/Remedial attempts)

Subject's name: Date:

Age:

Gender: Male/Female

Does the subject use spectacles? Yes/No

If yes, then mention type and power of spectacle lenses:

    Type of lens: Convex/Concave/Bifocal/Cylindrical

    Power of lens: Left side = _____ Dioptres.

              Right side = _____ Dioptres.

		Left eye	*Right eye*
Tests for Visual Acuity			
Distant vision*			
Near vision*			
*(*if the subject wears spectacles, it should be mentioned with the results.* *Example, visual acuity is 6/6 in left eye with spectacles.)*			
Ishihara's Tests for Colour Vision			
*No. of colour plates read correctly**			
Tests for Field of Vision			
Confrontation test *(mention whether normal/restricted in any quadrant)*			
Perimetry *(mention the field of vision in degrees in all quadrants).*	Superior Inferior Temporal Nasal	_____ degrees _____ degrees _____ degrees _____ degrees	_____ degrees _____ degrees _____ degrees _____ degrees

Result/Interpretation:

a. Visual Acuity

b. Colour vision

c. Field of vision

Signature of student   **Signature of teacher**

Note: Interpretation of Ishihara's tests

Out of initial 21 plates, if 17 or more plates are read correctly by an individual, then his colour sense should be regarded as normal. If 13 or less plates are read correctly, then the person has a red-green colour defect. Plates 22–25 are used for differential diagnosis of protans and deutans.

(*Ref:* Parmar T, Vananthi M, Ghose S, Dada T, Venkatesh P. Colour vision revisited. Delhi J Opthalmol 2014; 24(4):223–228.)

ASSESSMENT CARD FOR PROCEDURE 10*

Type of Attempt *(please tick):* **First/Repeat 1/Repeat 2/Remedial**
(use Xerox copy for Repeat/Remedial attempts)

Sr. No.	Attributes to be assessed	Score (1–5)*
i.	Behavioural skill	
ii.	Communication skill	
iii.	Confidence level	
iv.	Procedural skill	
v.	Knowledge level	
	Cumulative total (out of 25)	

*Note: The teacher may decide the score as given below:

Below average	Average	Good	Very good	Excellent
1	2	3	4	5

Grading of candidate (please tick): **B / M / E**

Cumulative total	Grading
9 or less	Below Expectations (B)
10–19	Meets Expectations (M)
20 and above	Exceeds Expectations (E)

Teacher's feedback:

_____

_____

_____

_____

_____

Signature of teacher (with date)

PROCEDURE 11

AIM: PY 10.20 Demonstrate hearing tests in a normal volunteer or simulated environment.

Number of times this skill needs to be done to be certified for independent performance = 01.

Sr. No.	Steps to be performed sequentially	Performed (Y/N)
	Checklist for procedure	
i.	Explains the procedure to the subject in his/her own language and double checks that the subject has fully understood the procedure.	
ii.	Ensures that there is no/minimum background noise in the room.	
iii.	Asks the subject to close his/her eyes and to focus on auditory stimulus with full concentration.	
iv.	Elicits whisper test.	
v.	Selects 256 Hz tuning fork.	
vi.	Performs Rinne's test.	
	a. Checks for bone conduction first by placing vibrating tuning fork on mastoid process of subject. b. As soon as subject lifts his/her finger, immediately keeps the tuning fork in front of subject's ear to check for air conduction.	
vii.	Performs Weber's test.	
	a. Keeps the vibrating tuning fork on forehead/vertex of subject's skull. b. Asks the subject if there is lateralisation of sound towards any ear.	
viii.	Performs Schwabach's test.	
	a. Places vibrating tuning fork initially on subjects mastoid process and then on his own mastoid process to compare bone conduction. b. Repeats the procedure to confirm the results by placing the vibrating tuning fork initially on his own mastoid process and thereafter on subject's mastoid process.	
ix.	Compares the result on both sides and records the findings in proper format.	

ACTIVITY PERFORMA FOR PROCEDURE 11

(use Xerox copy for Repeat/Remedial attempts)

Subject's name: Date:

Age:

Gender: Male/Female

Does the subject use hearing aids: Yes/No

If yes, then for which ear: Left ear/Right ear/Both ears

Hearing Tests Assessment

Tests performed	Left ear	Right ear
1. Whisper test (normal/abnormal)		
2. Tuning fork tests		
a. Rinne's test (AC>BC or AC<BC)		
b. Weber's test (not lateralised or lateralised towards…)		
c. Schwabach's test (BC of subject is equal to/ more than/less than examiner)		

Result/Interpretation:

Signature of student   **Signature of teacher**

ASSESSMENT CARD FOR PROCEDURE 11*

Type of Attempt (please tick): **First/Repeat 1/Repeat 2/Remedial**
(use Xerox copy for Repeat/Remedial attempts)

Sr. No.	Attributes to be assessed	Score (1–5)*
i.	Behavioural skill.	
ii.	Communication skill.	
iii.	Confidence level.	
iv.	Procedural skill.	
v.	Knowledge level.	
	Cumulative total (out of 25)	

*Note: The teacher may decide the score as given below:

Below average	Average	Good	Very good	Excellent
1	2	3	4	5

Grading of candidate (please tick): **B / M / E**

Cumulative total	Grading
9 or less	Below Expectations (B)
10–19	Meets Expectations (M)
20 and above	Exceeds Expectations (E)

Teacher's feedback:

_____

_____

_____

_____

_____

Signature of teacher (with date)

PROCEDURE 12

AIM: PY 10.20 Demonstrate testing of smell in a normal volunteer or simulated environment.

Number of times this skill needs to be done to be certified for independent performance = 01.

Checklist for procedure		
Sr. No.	Steps to be performed sequentially	Performed (Y/N)
i.	Explains the procedure to the subject in his/her own language.	
ii.	Checks that the nostrils are patent by compressing one nostril and asking the subject to sniff through the other.	
iii.	Asks the subject to close his/her eyes and also occlude opposite nostril.	
iv.	Keeps first odorant solution within 3 cm of one nostril of the subject.	
v.	Asks the subject to continuously sniff the solution for 3 seconds and identify it.	
vi.	Repeats the procedure with same odorant for other nostril.	
vii.	Repeats the procedure with another odorant sample after an interval of 30 seconds.	

Ref: Ferdenzi C, Poncelet J, Rouby C and Bensafi M (2014). Repeated exposure to odors induces affective habituation of perception and sniffing. Front. Behav. Neurosci. 8:119. doi: 10.3389/fnbeh.2014.00119

ACTIVITY PERFORMA FOR PROCEDURE 12

(use Xerox copy for Repeat/Remedial attempts)

Subject's name: Date:

Age:

Gender: Male/Female

Any history of allergy/rhinitis/persistent nasal blockade: Yes/No

Is the subject having common cold: Yes/No

Tests for Olfactory Perception
(*Results to be reported as perceived/not perceived)

Odorant used	Left nostril	Right nostril
1. Peppermint oil		
2. Clove oil		
3. Any other _____ (please specify)		

Result/Interpretation:

Signature of student   **Signature of teacher**

ASSESSMENT CARD FOR PROCEDURE 12*

Type of Attempt *(please tick):* **First/Repeat 1/Repeat 2/Remedial**
(use Xerox copy for Repeat/Remedial attempts)

Sr. No.	Attributes to be assessed	Score (1–5)*
i.	Behavioural skill	
ii.	Communication skill	
iii.	Confidence level	
iv.	Procedural skill	
v.	Knowledge level	
	Cumulative total (out of 25)	

*Note: The teacher may decide the score as given below:

Below average	Average	Good	Very good	Excellent
1	2	3	4	5

Grading of candidate (please tick): **B / M / E**

Cumulative total	Grading
9 or less	Below Expectations (B)
10–19	Meets Expectations (M)
20 and above	Exceeds Expectations (E)

Teacher's feedback:

_____

_____

_____

_____

_____

Signature of teacher (with date)

PROCEDURE 13

AIM: PY 10.20 Demonstrate taste sensation in a normal volunteer or simulated environment.

Number of times this skill needs to be done to be certified for independent performance = 01.

Sr. No.	Steps to be performed sequentially	Performed (Y/N)
	Checklist for procedure	
i.	Explains the procedure to the subject in his/her own language.	
ii.	Asks the subject not to speak during the test.	
iii.	Provides him four cards to indicate the names of the perceived taste.	
iv.	Asks the subject to thoroughly rinse his/her mouth before starting the procedure.	
v.	Asks the subject to close his/her eyes and also protrude his tongue.	
vi.	With a dropper, pours a few drops of a taste solution on anterior 2/3rds of tongue.	
vii.	Asks the subject to indicate the taste perceived by picking up the corresponding card indicating the name of that taste.	
viii.	Ensures that the subject rinses his/her mouth thoroughly before putting a new taste solution on his/her tongue.	
ix.	Tests for the remaining taste sensations in a similar manner.	
x.	Tests the bitter sensation at the end.	

ACTIVITY PERFORMA FOR PROCEDURE 13

(use Xerox copy for Repeat/Remedial attempts)

Subject's name: Date:

Age:

Gender: Male/Female

Tests for Gustatory Perception

Taste sample	Findings (Perceived/Not perceived)
1. Sweet solution	
2. Salt solution	
3. Sour solution	
4. Bitter solution	

Result/Interpretation:

Signature of student   **Signature of teacher**

ASSESSMENT CARD FOR PROCEDURE 13*
Type of Attempt *(please tick)*: **First/Repeat 1/Repeat 2/Remedial**
(use Xerox copy for Repeat/Remedial attempts)

Sr. No.	Attributes to be assessed	Score (1–5)*
i.	Behavioural skill	
ii.	Communication skill	
iii.	Confidence level	
iv.	Procedural skill	
v.	Knowledge level	
	Cumulative total (out of 25)	

Note: The teacher may decide the score as given below:

Below average	Average	Good	Very good	Excellent
1	2	3	4	5

Grading of candidate (please tick): **B / M / E**

Cumulative total	Grading
9 or less	Below Expectations (B)
10–19	Meets Expectations (M)
20 and above	Exceeds Expectations (E)

Teacher's feedback:

_____

_____

_____

_____

_____

Signature of teacher (with date)

Notes

Notes

Notes

Notes

Notes

Notes

Notes

Notes

Notes

Notes

Notes

Notes

Certificate of Completion

This is to certify that Mr/Ms _____ Registration no. _____ admitted in the year 20___ –20___

in _____ Medical College, _____ has satisfactorily completed/ has not completed all the

13 clinical competencies mentioned in this logbook for First year MBBS course in the subject of Physiology during the

period from _____ to _____. He/she is eligible/ineligible to appear for the summative (University) assessment

as on the date given below.

Signature of faculty in-charge

Name: _____

Designation: _____

Countersigned by

Head of the Department

Principal/Dean of the College

Place:

Date: